FAST LIKE A GIRL DIET COOKBOOK

Unlocking Fat-Burning, Energizing, and Hormone-Balancing Secrets for Women

Lori J. Garcia

Table Of Contents

Introduction 6

CHAPTER 1: THE HEALING POWER OF FASTING 10

Understanding the Female Body: Hormones, Metabolism, and Fasting 11

How Fasting Promotes Fat Burning, Energy Boosting, and Hormone Balance 13

Menstrual Cycle Considerations 15

Pregnancy, Postpartum, and Fasting 18

CHAPTER 3: ENERGIZING BREAKFASTS 21

Chia Seed Pudding with Berries 21

Avocado and Smoked Salmon Toast 22

Greek Yogurt Parfait 23

Spinach and Feta Omelette 24

Quinoa Breakfast Bowl 25

Smoothie Bowl with Greens 25

Turmeric and Ginger Oatmeal 26

Cottage Cheese and Pineapple Bowl 27

Coconut and Almond Flour Pancakes 28

Mango and Coconut Chia Pudding 29

CHAPTER 4: NOURISHING LUNCHES 31

Grilled Chicken Salad with Avocado 31

Quinoa and Chickpea Buddha Bowl 32

Salmon and Asparagus Stir-Fry 33

Mushroom and Spinach Quiche 34

Sweet Potato and Black Bean Bowl 35

Lentil and Vegetable Soup 36

Turkey and Quinoa Stuffed Bell Peppers 37

Eggplant and Chickpea Curry 38

Shrimp and Quinoa Salad 39

Chicken and Broccoli Stir-Fry with Brown

Rice 40

CHAPTER 5: SATISFYING DINNERS 42

Salmon and Quinoa Stuffed Bell Peppers 43

Vegetarian Zucchini Noodles with Pesto 44

Turkey and Sweet Potato Skillet 45

Mushroom and Spinach Stuffed Chicken

Breast 46

Lentil and Vegetable Stir-Fry with Tofu 47

Egg Fried Cauliflower Rice with Shrimp 48

Chickpea and Vegetable Curry 49

Stuffed Portobello Mushrooms with Quinoa and

Feta 50

Sesame Ginger Tofu Stir-Fry with Brown

Rice 51

Cauliflower Alfredo with Grilled Chicken 52

CHAPTER 6: DELICIOUS SNACKS AND

TREATS 54

Greek Yogurt Parfait with Berries and

Almonds 55

Cucumber and Hummus Bites 56

Energy-Boosting Trail Mix 57

Apple Slices with Almond Butter 58

Coconut and Almond Bliss Balls 58

Chia Seed Pudding with Mango 59

Yogurt-Dipped Strawberries 60

Avocado and Tomato Salsa 61

Frozen Banana Bites 62

Pumpkin Spice Smoothie Bowl 63

CHAPTER 7: DELICIOUS DESSERT 64

Chocolate Avocado Mousse 90

Berry and Yogurt Parfait 91

Pumpkin Chia Seed Pudding 92

Coconut and Almond Flour Brownies 93

Mango Sorbet 94

Baked Apples with Cinnamon and Walnuts 94

Cherry Almond Dark Chocolate Bark 95

Blueberry Lemon Cheesecake Bites 96

Banana and Peanut Butter Ice Cream 97

Lemon Poppy Seed Yogurt Cake 98

CHAPTER 8: FASTING LIKE A GIRL

WORKBOOK 65

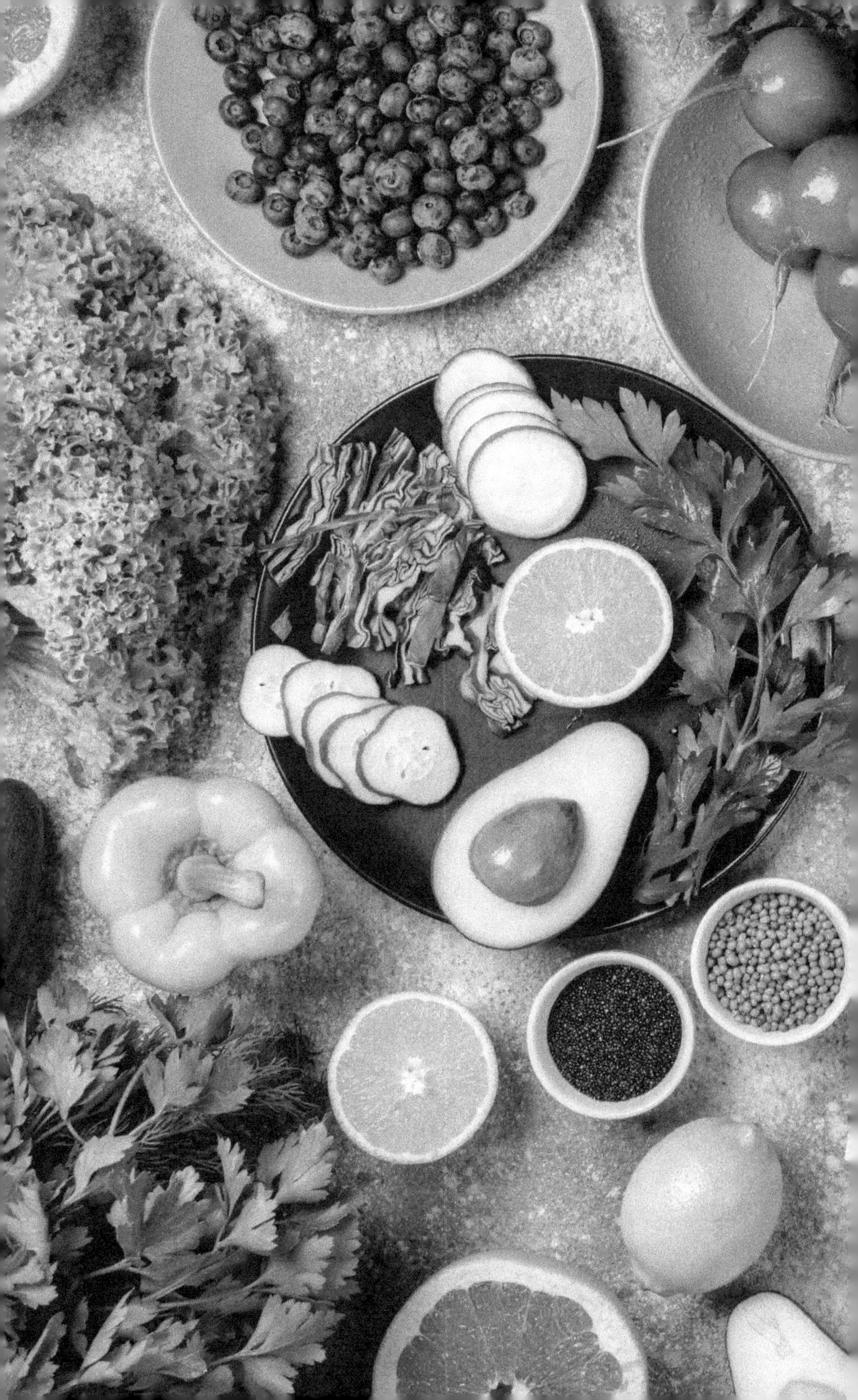

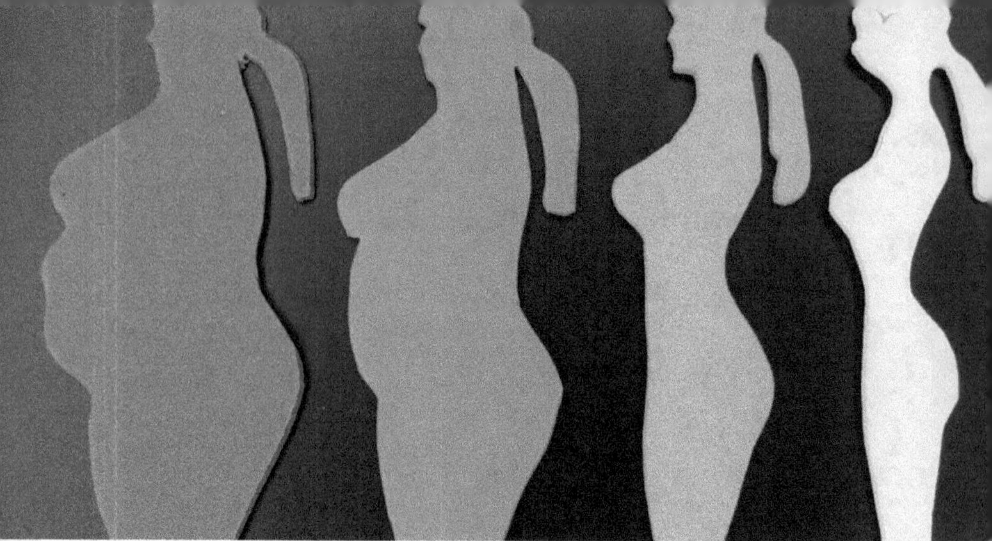

INTRODUCTION

In the bustling city of empowerment, where women seek not just physical strength but a holistic approach to health, a revolutionary guide has emerged – "Fast Like a Girl Diet Cookbook." Within its pages lies a transformative journey tailored for women who are ready to redefine their relationship with food, harness the healing power of fasting, and embrace a lifestyle that champions strength, energy, and hormonal balance.

Meet Sarah, a modern woman navigating the challenges of a fast-paced life, juggling career ambitions, family responsibilities, and personal well-being. Frustrated by the one-size-fits-all approach to dieting and wellness, Sarah stumbled upon the Fast Like a Girl philosophy. Intrigued, she embarked on a journey that would not only transform her body but also reshape her understanding of what it means to be fast, fierce, and female.

The introduction of this groundbreaking guide immerses readers in Sarah's story, providing a relatable entry point for women from all walks of life. Through her experiences, doubts, and triumphs, the narrative unfolds, seamlessly connecting with the reader's own struggles and aspirations. The book becomes a trusted companion, understanding the nuances of a woman's body, acknowledging the uniqueness of her hormonal landscape, and presenting a path to wellness that goes beyond superficial weight loss.

As Sarah delves into the pages of the "Fast Like a Girl Diet Cookbook," she discovers not just a collection of recipes but a comprehensive roadmap. The book unfolds with chapters on the science behind fasting for women, practical tips for getting started, diverse fasting protocols, and an enticing array of recipes tailored for the feminine palate. Each page is infused with a commitment to fostering a healthy mind-body connection, encouraging mindful eating, and incorporating tailored workouts designed for women.

Through seasonal adaptations, stress management strategies, and insightful anecdotes from women who have embraced the Fast Like a Girl lifestyle, the guide becomes a beacon of support for readers navigating their own unique journeys. The introduction sets the stage for a transformative experience, inviting women to reclaim control over their bodies, boost their energy, and find harmony in hormonal balance.

"Fast Like a Girl Diet Cookbook" isn't just a book; it's a celebration of the feminine spirit, a guide to unleashing the inherent strength within, and a roadmap to living life unapologetically, fast and fierce, just like a girl. Join Sarah and countless others as they embark on a transformative journey towards a healthier, more empowered version of themselves.

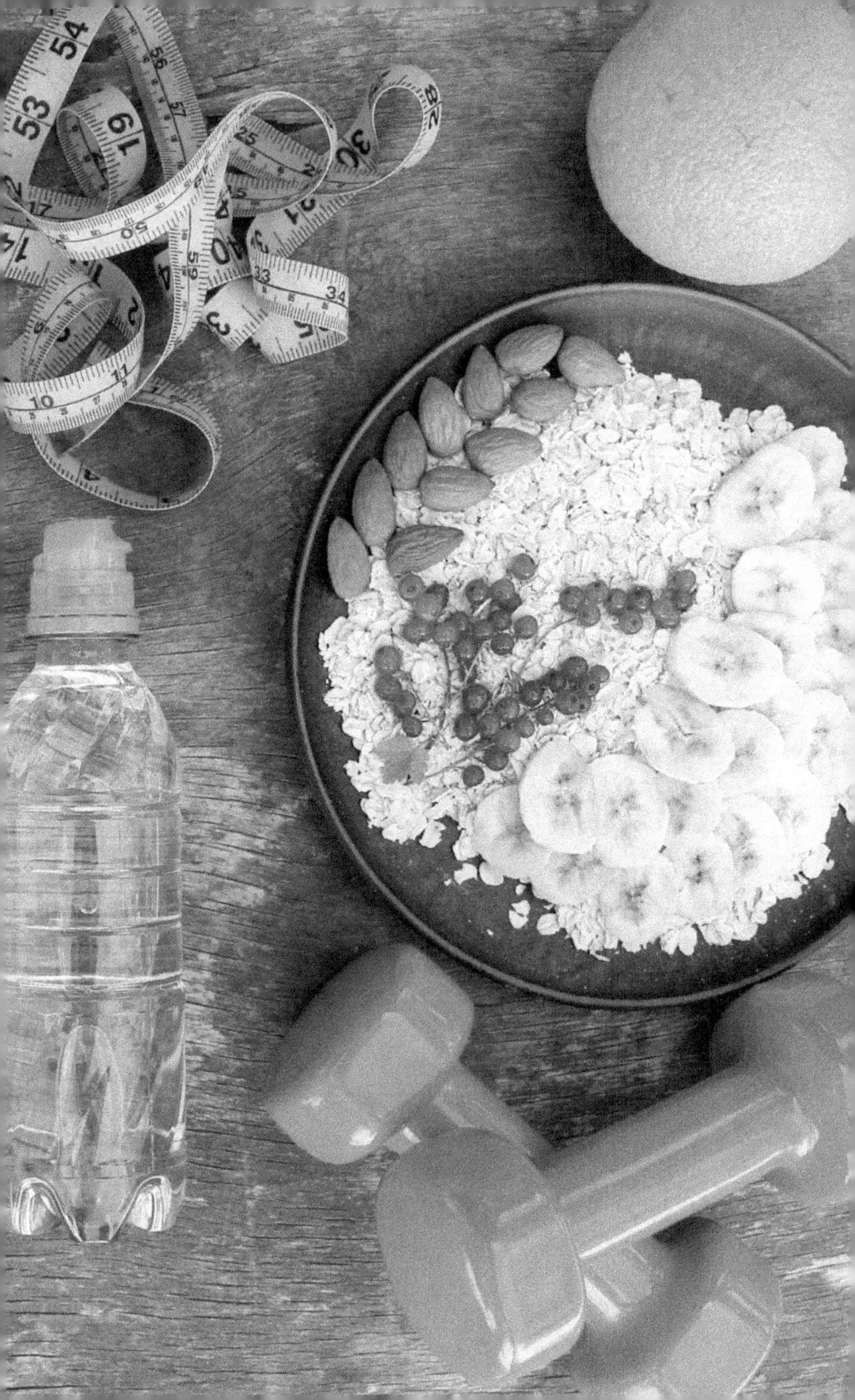

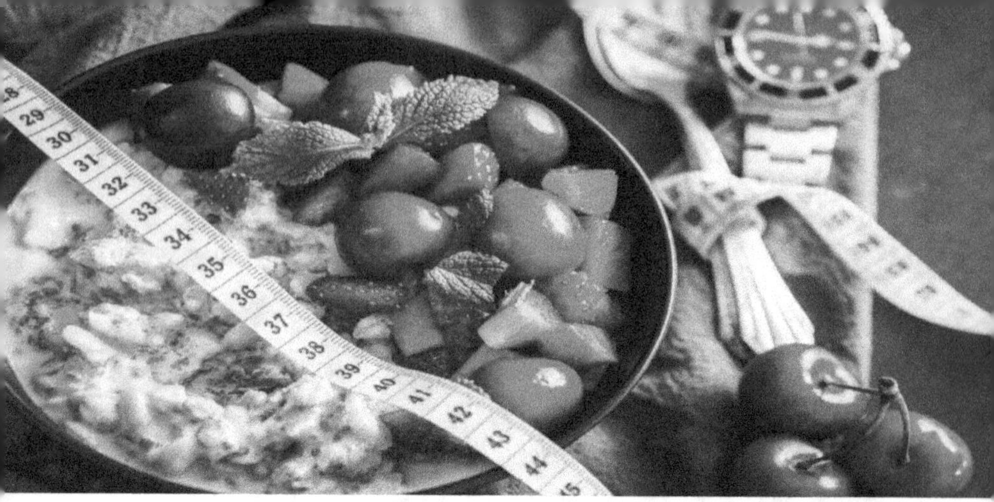

CHAPTER 1: THE HEALING POWER OF FASTING

Understanding the Female Body: Hormones, Metabolism, and Fasting

The Dance of Hormones:

Delving into the complex hormonal symphony that orchestrates a woman's body, this section unveils the pivotal roles played by estrogen, progesterone, and other hormones in shaping health and well-being. It explores the cyclical nature of the menstrual cycle, offering insights into how fasting can complement and support hormonal balance. Readers embark on a journey to understand how fasting can positively influence mood, energy levels, and the overall ebb and flow of hormones throughout the month.

Metabolic Mastery:

Unveiling the intricacies of a woman's metabolism, this segment provides a roadmap for navigating the unique metabolic pathways that define female physiology. It explores how fasting can become a powerful ally in optimizing metabolic health, enhancing insulin sensitivity, and unlocking the body's innate ability to burn fat efficiently. Through this understanding, women gain the tools to customize their fasting practices, ensuring alignment with their metabolic needs and goals.

Fasting Through Life's Phases:

Acknowledging the dynamic nature of a woman's life journey, this section navigates through various stages, from adolescence to menopause and beyond. It offers tailored insights on how fasting can be adapted to the specific needs of women during puberty, fertility, pregnancy, postpartum, and the transitions of menopause. Recognizing that the female body evolves, the chapter becomes a reliable guide for embracing fasting as a lifelong companion through different phases of life.

Beyond the physical, this chapter underscores the intimate connection between the female body and mind. It explores how fasting can influence cognitive function, mental clarity, and emotional well-being. By understanding this mind-body synergy, women are empowered to embrace fasting not just as a tool for physical health but as a holistic practice that nurtures mental resilience and emotional balance.

How Fasting Promotes Fat Burning, Energy Boosting, and Hormone Balance

Igniting Fat Burning Furnaces:

The journey into fat burning begins with a profound exploration of how fasting serves as the key to unlocking the body's natural ability to burn fat efficiently. As the body enters a fasting state, it shifts from relying on readily available glucose to tapping into stored fat reserves. This metabolic switch not only aids in shedding excess fat but also promotes a sustainable and long-term approach to weight management.

Unleashing Energy Reservoirs:

Central to the fasting narrative is the revelation of how this practice becomes a catalyst for an unparalleled energy boost. As the body transitions into a fasted state, cellular mechanisms are activated to enhance mitochondrial function. This heightened efficiency in energy production translates into increased vitality, mental clarity, and a sustained source of energy that transcends the fleeting spikes induced by conventional eating patterns.

Harmonizing Hormones for Women:

At the heart of this exploration is the intricate dance between fasting and hormonal balance. Fasting has the remarkable ability to modulate key hormones such as insulin, estrogen, and ghrelin, contributing to a harmonious hormonal milieu. By stabilizing blood sugar levels and reducing insulin resistance, fasting emerges as a powerful tool for managing weight, improving insulin sensitivity, and mitigating the risk of hormonal imbalances that can impact reproductive health and overall well-being.

Resetting the Circadian Rhythm:

Fasting becomes a conductor orchestrating the symphony of the body's internal clock, the circadian rhythm. By aligning eating patterns with the natural circadian cycle, fasting optimizes hormonal secretion, enhances metabolic efficiency, and contributes to a sense of overall balance. This nuanced understanding allows women to synchronize their fasting practices with their body's internal rhythm, fostering a holistic approach to health.

Beyond fat burning, energy enhancement, and hormonal equilibrium, fasting emerges as a potent ally in the fight against inflammation and oxidative stress. Through mechanisms like autophagy, fasting encourages cellular repair and regeneration, contributing to a reduction in inflammation and bolstering the body's resilience against the detrimental effects of oxidative stress.

Tailoring Fasting to Women's Unique Needs

Menstrual Cycle Considerations

Menstrual Phase:

The chapter begins by acknowledging the menstrual phase, a time when women may experience hormonal shifts, changes in energy levels, and varying emotional states. Fasting during this phase may involve gentle modifications to accommodate the body's natural need for nourishment and support. By understanding these cyclical changes, women can adjust their fasting patterns to foster self-compassion and alignment with the body's inherent wisdom.

Follicular Phase:

As the body transitions into the follicular phase, marked by the end of menstruation, fasting practices can adapt to the rising levels of estrogen. This phase often coincides with an increase in energy and vitality, making it an opportune time for more intensive fasting if desired. Insights into optimizing nutrient intake and energy expenditure during this period contribute to a holistic approach that complements the body's natural state.

Ovulatory Phase:

Fasting during the ovulatory phase, characterized by the release of the egg and a surge in estrogen, can align with the body's heightened metabolic state. This phase offers an opportunity to explore fasting strategies that support energy levels, cognitive function, and physical performance. Understanding the body's inherent strengths during this phase allows women to harness the benefits of fasting more effectively.

Luteal Phase:

As the luteal phase unfolds, accompanied by a rise in progesterone, considerations for energy levels and potential cravings come to the forefront. Tailoring fasting practices to address these fluctuations becomes paramount, emphasizing nutrient-dense meals to support overall well-being. Acknowledging the body's needs during this phase fosters a compassionate and sustainable approach to fasting.

Holistic Wellness throughout the Cycle:

The chapter weaves these considerations into a tapestry of holistic wellness, encouraging women to view their menstrual cycle as a guide rather than a hindrance. By aligning fasting practices with the natural fluctuations in hormones, women can embrace a more personalized and empowering approach to health. This nuanced understanding not only optimizes the benefits of fasting but also cultivates a deeper connection with one's body.

Pregnancy, Postpartum, and Fasting

Pregnancy:

As the chapter opens its pages to the miracle of pregnancy, it does so with reverence, recognizing the profound changes a woman's body undergoes to nurture new life. Fasting during pregnancy becomes a gentle exploration, emphasizing the importance of nourishment and mindful eating. The focus shifts from restrictive fasting to embracing nutrient-dense meals that support the growing baby and provide the necessary energy for the mother. It is a chapter that encourages a connection with the body's wisdom, fostering a holistic approach that prioritizes the well-being of both mother and child.

Postpartum:

The journey through postpartum unfolds with a tender acknowledgment of the physical and emotional recovery after childbirth. Fasting, in this phase, transforms into a practice of self-care and nurturing. It involves adapting to the evolving needs of the body, allowing time for healing, and embracing a gradual return to fasting practices. The chapter provides insights into nourishing meals that aid recovery, recognizing that the postpartum period is a delicate balance of self-love, restoration, and embracing the joys of new motherhood.

Fasting as a Personal Journey:

Interwoven within these chapters is the realization that fasting is not a rigid set of rules but a deeply personal journey. It becomes a tool for self-discovery, a way for mothers to reconnect with their bodies, and a means of finding balance amidst the beautiful chaos of raising a child. Fasting during pregnancy and postpartum is not about perfection but about navigating each day with intention, flexibility, and a gentle understanding of one's own needs.

Nurturing the Mother-Child Bond:

The chapter emphasizes the importance of nurturing the mother-child bond through mindful practices. Fasting becomes a shared experience, a rhythm that echoes between mother and child. It involves savoring moments of nourishment, cherishing the act of feeding, and embracing the shared journey of growth and development.

Compassionate Adaptation:

Above all, "Pregnancy, Postpartum, and Fasting" is a testament to the strength and resilience of women. It advocates for a compassionate adaptation of fasting practices, understanding that every pregnancy and postpartum experience is unique. It encourages mothers to listen to their bodies, seek support when needed, and embrace a fluid approach to fasting that aligns with the ever-evolving tapestry of motherhood.

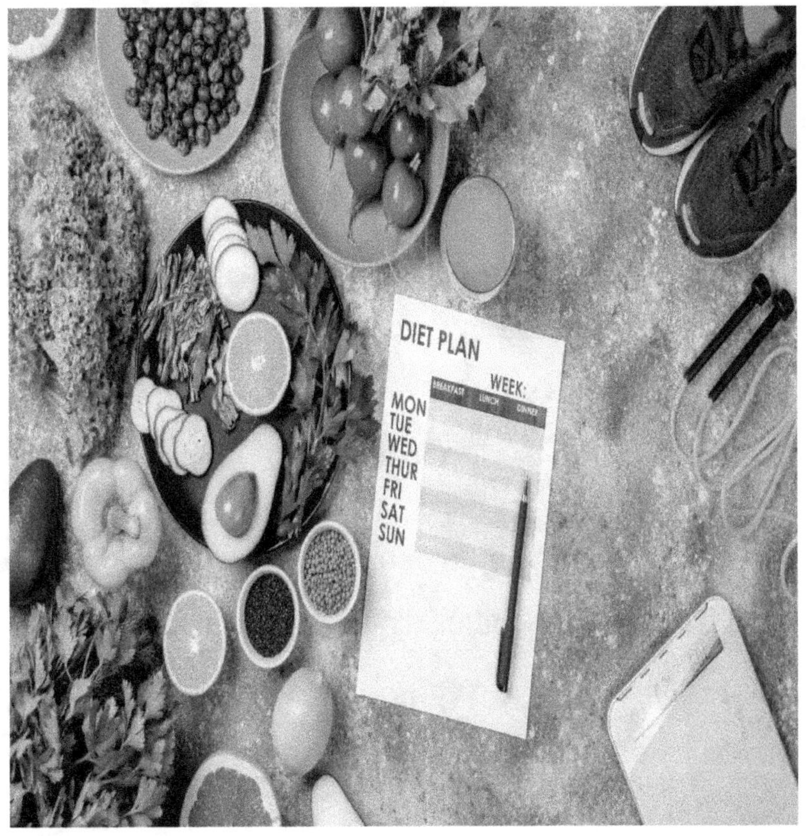

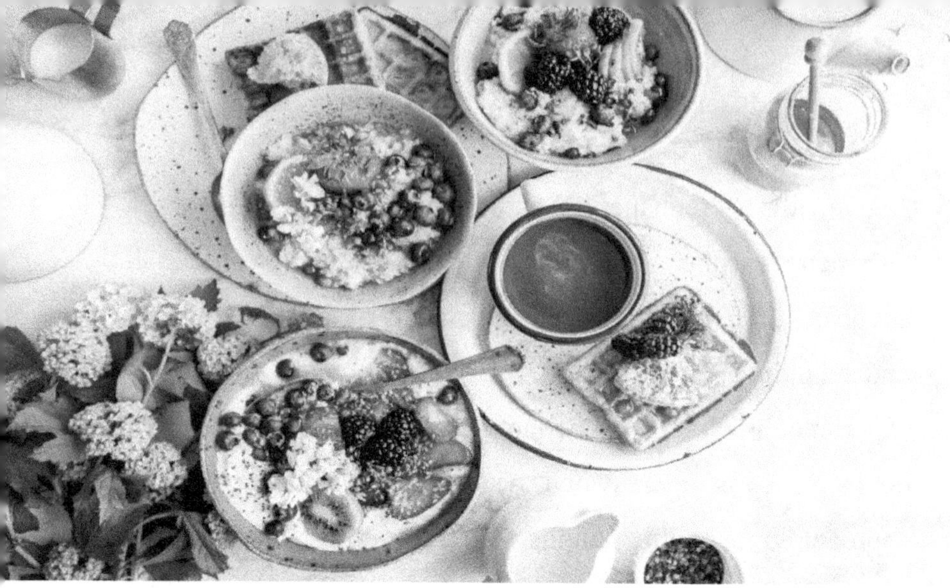

CHAPTER 3: ENERGIZING BREAKFASTS

Chia Seed Pudding with Berries

Ingredients:

- 1/4 cup chia seeds

- 1 cup almond milk

- 1/2 teaspoon vanilla extract

- Mixed berries (blueberries, strawberries, raspberries)

Instructions:

1. Mix chia seeds, almond milk, and vanilla extract in a bowl.
2. Refrigerate overnight or for at least 4 hours.
3. Top with mixed berries before serving.

Prep Time: *5 minutes (plus chilling time)*
Chia seeds provide omega-3 fatty acids and fiber, promoting satiety and hormonal balance.

Avocado and Smoked Salmon Toast

Ingredients:

- 1 slice whole-grain bread
- 1/2 ripe avocado
- Smoked salmon slices
- Lemon juice
- Dill for garnish

Instructions:

1. Toast the bread to your liking.
2. Mash the avocado and spread it on the toast.

3. Arrange smoked salmon on top, drizzle with lemon juice, and garnish with dill.

Prep Time: *10 minutes*

Avocado offers healthy fats, and smoked salmon provides omega-3 fatty acids for brain health and hormonal support.

Greek Yogurt Parfait

Ingredients:

- 1 cup Greek yogurt
- 1/2 cup granola
- Mixed fresh fruits (such as berries and mango)

Instructions:

1. In a glass or bowl, layer Greek yogurt, granola, and mixed fruits.
2. Repeat the layers until the container is filled.

Prep Time: *5 minutes*

Greek yogurt is rich in protein and probiotics, supporting gut health and hormonal balance.

Spinach and Feta Omelette

Ingredients:

- 2 eggs
- Handful of fresh spinach
- 1/4 cup feta cheese
- Salt and pepper to taste

Instructions:

1. Whisk eggs in a bowl and season with salt and pepper.
2. Sauté spinach in a pan until wilted.
3. Pour eggs over spinach, add feta, and cook until set.

Prep Time: *10 minutes*

Eggs provide essential amino acids, while spinach offers iron and feta contributes calcium.

Quinoa Breakfast Bowl

Ingredients:

- 1/2 cup cooked quinoa
- 1/4 cup sliced almonds
- 1/2 cup mixed berries
- Drizzle of honey

Instructions:

1. Combine cooked quinoa, sliced almonds, and mixed berries in a bowl.
2. Drizzle with honey before serving.

Prep Time: *15 minutes*

Quinoa is a complete protein source, and almonds provide healthy fats and vitamin E.

Smoothie Bowl with Greens

Ingredients:

- 1 cup spinach or kale

- 1/2 frozen banana
- 1/2 cup frozen berries
- 1/2 cup almond milk
- Toppings: granola, chia seeds, sliced fruit

Instructions:

1. Blend spinach, banana, berries, and almond milk until smooth.
2. Pour into a bowl and top with granola, chia seeds, and sliced fruit.

Prep Time: *5 minutes*

Leafy greens offer vitamins and minerals, while the smoothie provides a nutrient-packed start.

Turmeric and Ginger Oatmeal

Ingredients:

- 1/2 cup rolled oats
- 1 cup almond milk
- 1/2 teaspoon turmeric

- 1/2 teaspoon grated ginger
- Toppings: sliced banana, walnuts

Instructions:

1. Cook oats with almond milk, turmeric, and grated ginger.
2. Top with sliced banana and walnuts.

Prep Time: *10 minutes*

Turmeric and ginger have anti-inflammatory properties, and oats offer complex carbohydrates for sustained energy.

Cottage Cheese and Pineapple Bowl

Ingredients:

- 1 cup low-fat cottage cheese
- 1 cup fresh pineapple chunks
- 1 tablespoon flaxseeds

Instructions:

1. Combine cottage cheese and pineapple in a bowl.

2. Sprinkle flaxseeds on top before serving.

Prep Time: *5 minutes*

Cottage cheese provides protein and pineapple adds natural sweetness and vitamin C.

Coconut and Almond Flour Pancakes

Ingredients:

- 1/2 cup almond flour
- 2 tablespoons coconut flour
- 2 eggs
- 1/4 cup almond milk
- Toppings: Greek yogurt, sliced strawberries

Instructions:

1. Mix almond flour, coconut flour, eggs, and almond milk in a bowl.

2. Cook pancakes on a griddle.

3. Top with Greek yogurt and sliced strawberries.

Prep Time: *15 minutes*

Almond and coconut flours offer a gluten-free alternative with healthy fats.

Mango and Coconut Chia Pudding

Ingredients:

- 1/4 cup chia seeds
- 1 cup coconut milk
- 1/2 ripe mango, diced
- Shredded coconut for garnish

Instructions:

1. Mix chia seeds and coconut milk in a bowl.
2. Refrigerate until set, then layer with diced mango.
3. Garnish with shredded coconut.

Prep Time: *5 minutes (plus chilling time)*

Coconut milk provides healthy fats, and mango adds natural sweetness and vitamin C.

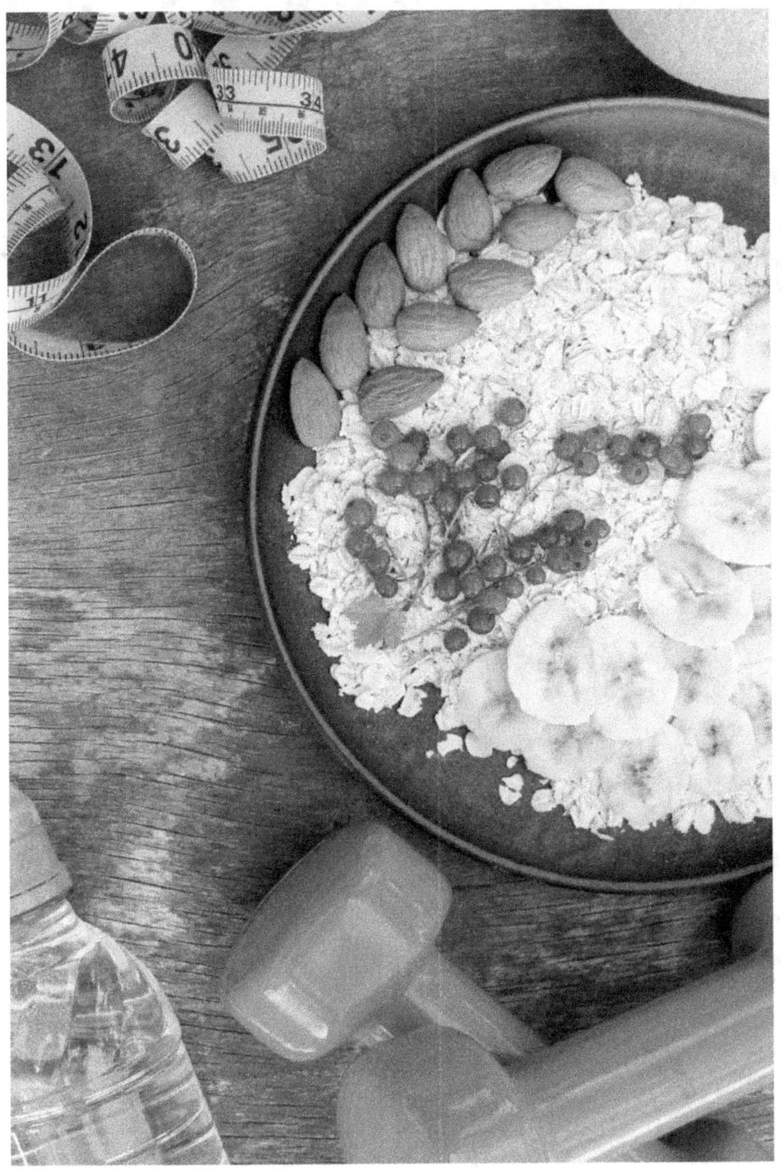

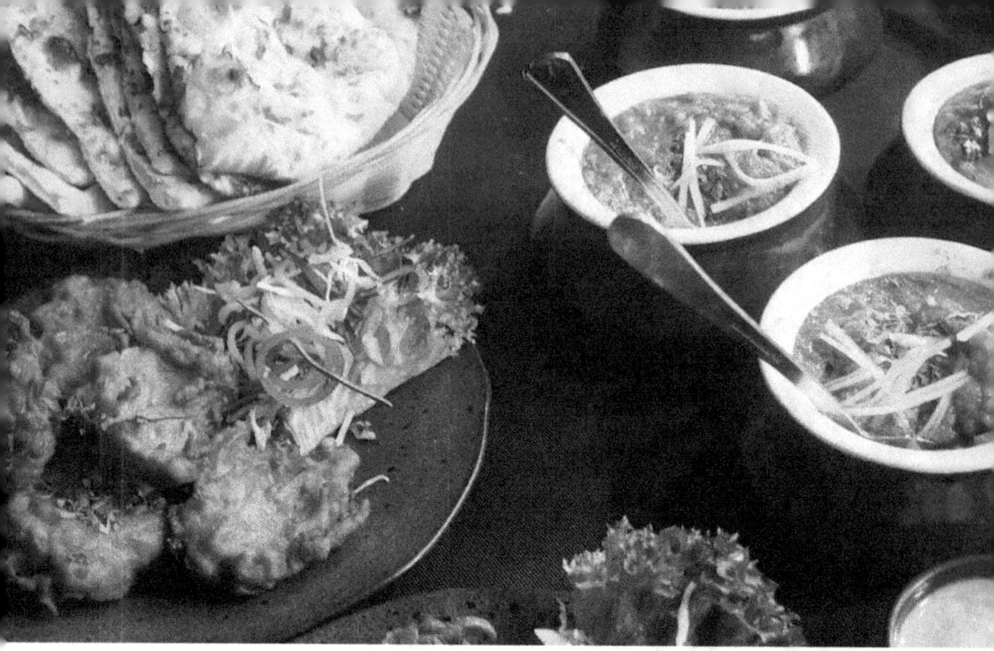

CHAPTER 4: NOURISHING LUNCHES

Grilled Chicken Salad with Avocado

Ingredients:

- grilled chicken breast
- Mixed salad greens
- Cherry tomatoes
- Cucumber slices
- Avocado slices
- Olive oil and balsamic vinegar dressing

1. Grill the chicken breast until fully cooked.

2. Combine salad greens, cherry tomatoes, cucumber slices, and avocado slices in a bowl.

3. Slice the grilled chicken and place it on top of the salad. Drizzle with olive oil and balsamic vinegar dressing.

Prep Time: *20 minutes*

Grilled chicken provides lean protein, while avocado adds healthy fats and a creamy texture.

Quinoa and Chickpea Buddha Bowl

Ingredients:

- 1/2 cup cooked quinoa
- 1/2 cup chickpeas (canned or cooked)
- Sliced bell peppers
- Shredded carrots
- Kale or spinach leaves

- Tahini dressing

Instructions:

1. Arrange quinoa, chickpeas, bell peppers, shredded carrots, and greens in a bowl.
2. Drizzle with tahini dressing before serving.

Prep Time: *15 minutes*

Quinoa and chickpeas combine to offer a plant-based protein powerhouse, and vegetables provide essential nutrients.

Salmon and Asparagus Stir-Fry

Ingredients:

- Salmon fillet
- Asparagus spears
- Bell peppers, thinly sliced
- Garlic, minced
- Soy sauce
- Sesame oil

1. Stir-fry salmon, asparagus, bell peppers, and garlic in sesame oil.
2. Add soy sauce for flavor.
3. Serve over a bed of brown rice or cauliflower rice.

Prep Time: *15 minutes*

Salmon provides omega-3 fatty acids, while asparagus and bell peppers contribute vitamins and fiber.

Mushroom and Spinach Quiche

Ingredients:

- Pie crust (store-bought or homemade)
- Eggs
- Milk or almond milk
- Mushrooms, sliced
- Fresh spinach

- Feta or goat cheese

Instructions:

1. Line the pie crust with mushrooms, fresh spinach, and cheese.
2. Whisk eggs with milk, pour over the vegetables and cheese.
3. Bake until the quiche is set and golden brown.

Prep Time: *30 minutes*

Eggs provide protein, and spinach and mushrooms offer vitamins and minerals.

Sweet Potato and Black Bean Bowl

Ingredients:

- Roasted sweet potatoes
- Black beans (canned or cooked)
- Corn kernels
- Cherry tomatoes, halved
- Avocado slices

- Lime dressing

Instructions:

1. Combine roasted sweet potatoes, black beans, corn, cherry tomatoes, and avocado in a bowl.
2. Drizzle with lime dressing before serving.

Prep Time: 25 minutes

Sweet potatoes are rich in complex carbohydrates, and black beans provide fiber and protein.

Lentil and Vegetable Soup

Ingredients:

- Lentils, rinsed
- Carrots, diced
- Celery, chopped
- Onion, finely chopped
- Vegetable broth
- Spinach leaves

1. In a pot, sauté onions, carrots, and celery until softened.
2. Add lentils and vegetable broth, then simmer until lentils are cooked.
3. Stir in spinach leaves before serving.

Prep Time: *30 minutes*

Lentils offer plant-based protein, and vegetables provide a range of vitamins and minerals.

Turkey and Quinoa Stuffed Bell Peppers

Ingredients:

- Bell peppers, halved
- Ground turkey
- Cooked quinoa
- Diced tomatoes
- Black beans (canned or cooked)
- Taco seasoning

1. Brown ground turkey and mix with cooked quinoa, diced tomatoes, black beans, and taco seasoning.
2. Stuff bell peppers with the turkey and quinoa mixture.
3. Bake until peppers are tender.

Prep Time: *40 minutes*

Turkey offers lean protein, and quinoa adds a complete protein source with essential amino acids.

Eggplant and Chickpea Curry

Ingredients:

- Eggplant, diced
- Chickpeas (canned or cooked)
- Coconut milk
- Curry powder
- Garlic, minced
- Basmati rice

1. Sauté eggplant, chickpeas, and minced garlic in a pan.

2. Add coconut milk and curry powder, simmer until eggplant is tender.

3. Serve over cooked basmati rice.

Prep Time: *35 minutes*

Eggplant provides fiber, and chickpeas offer plant-based protein and essential nutrients.

Shrimp and Quinoa Salad

Ingredients:

- Cooked shrimp
- Cooked quinoa
- Cherry tomatoes, halved
- Cucumber, diced
- Feta cheese
- Lemon vinaigrette

1. Combine cooked shrimp, quinoa, cherry tomatoes, cucumber, and feta cheese in a bowl.
2. Drizzle with lemon vinaigrette before serving.

Prep Time: *25 minutes*

Shrimp provides lean protein, and quinoa adds a nutrient-dense base to the salad.

Chicken and Broccoli Stir-Fry with Brown Rice

Ingredients:

- Chicken breast, thinly sliced
- Broccoli florets
- Carrots, julienned
- Soy sauce
- Ginger, minced
- Brown rice, cooked

1. Stir-fry chicken, broccoli, and carrots in soy sauce and minced ginger.

2. Serve over cooked brown rice.

Prep Time: *20 minutes*

Chicken offers lean protein, while broccoli and carrots provide essential vitamins and fiber.

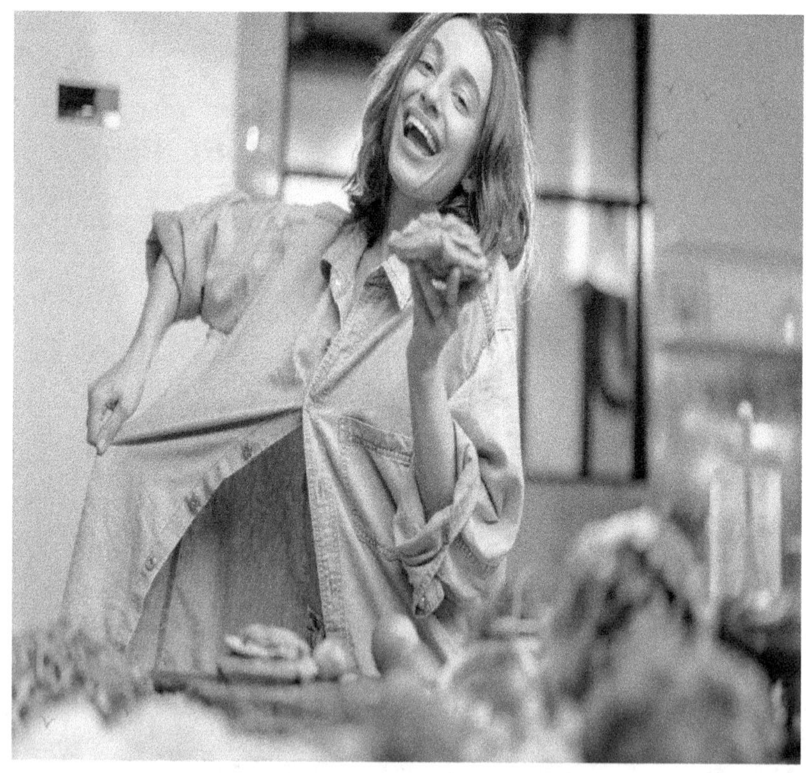

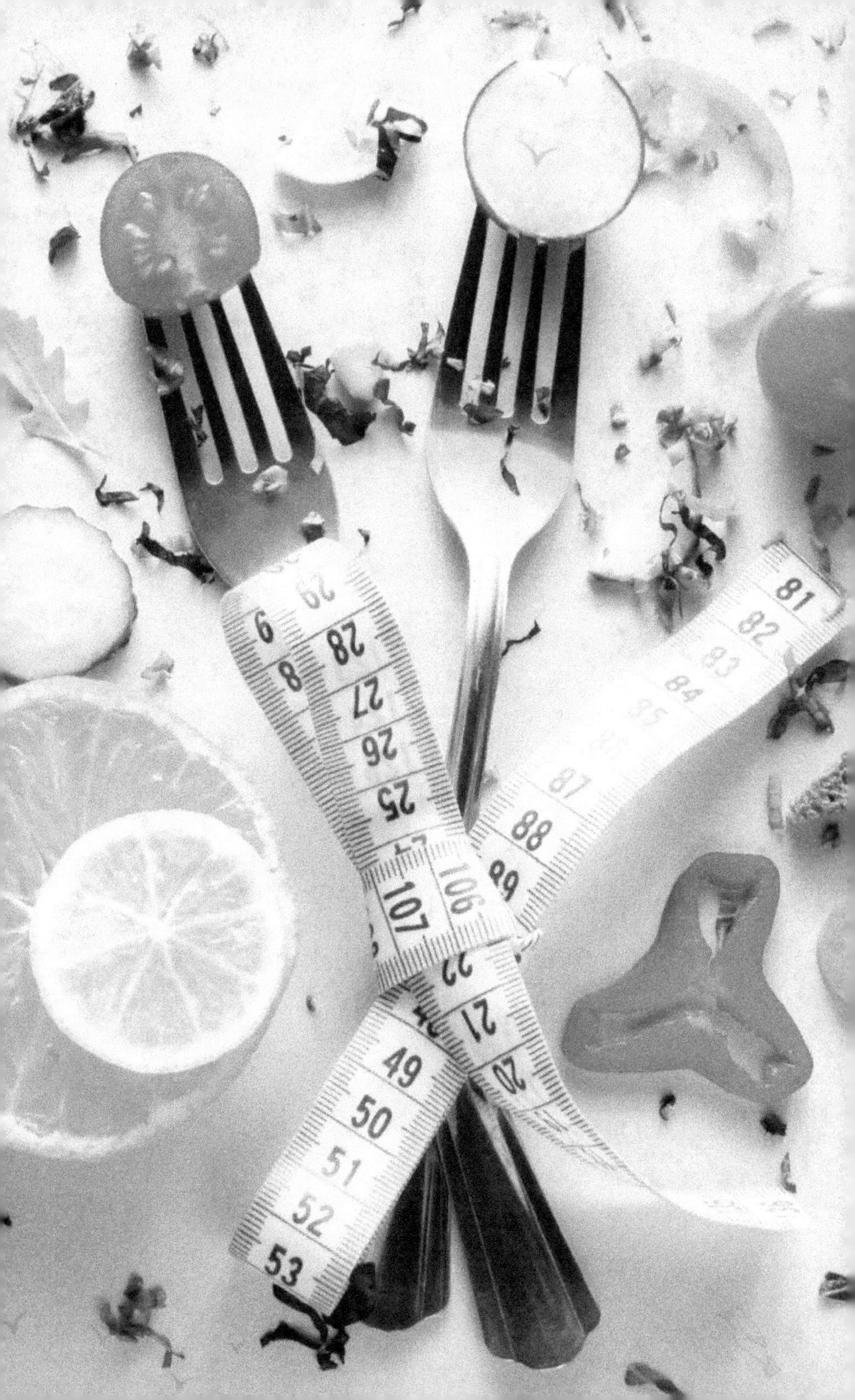

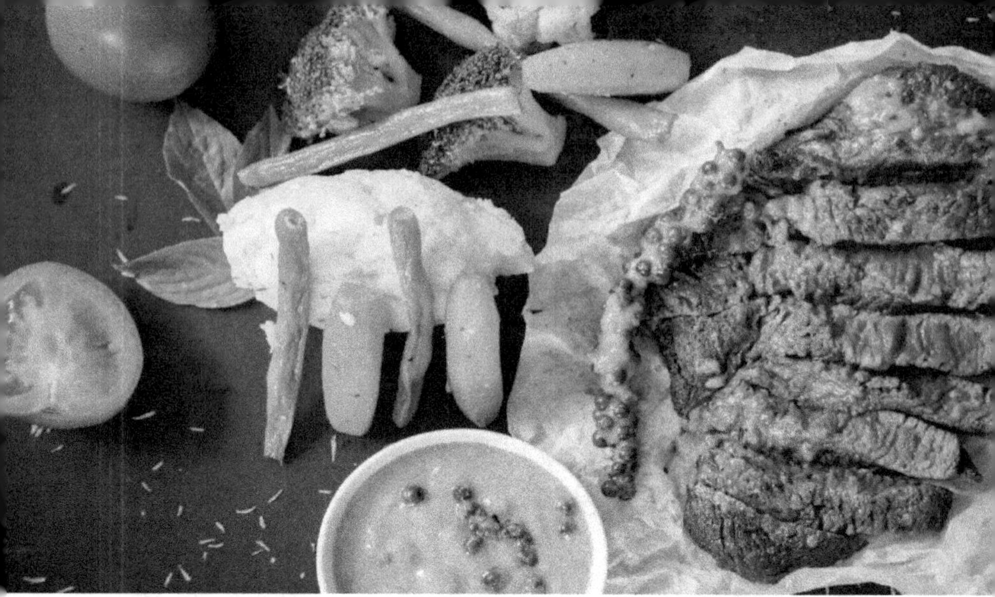

CHAPTER 5: SATISFYING DINNERS

Salmon and Quinoa Stuffed Bell Peppers

Ingredients:

- Bell peppers, halved
- Salmon fillet, cooked and flaked
- Cooked quinoa
- Spinach leaves
- Feta cheese
- Lemon zest

1. Mix flaked salmon, quinoa, spinach, and feta cheese.
2. Stuff bell peppers with the mixture.
3. Bake until peppers are tender. Garnish with lemon zest.

Prep Time: *30 minutes*

Salmon provides omega-3 fatty acids, while quinoa offers complete protein and fiber.

Vegetarian Zucchini Noodles with Pesto

Ingredients:

- Zucchini, spiralized
- Cherry tomatoes, halved
- Pine nuts
- Fresh basil pesto
- Parmesan cheese

Instructions:

1. Sauté zucchini noodles and cherry tomatoes.

2. Toss with pine nuts and fresh basil pesto.

3. Top with grated Parmesan cheese.

Prep Time: *20 minutes*

Zucchini is low in calories, and the pesto provides healthy fats and flavor.

Turkey and Sweet Potato Skillet

Ingredients:

- Ground turkey
- Sweet potatoes, diced
- Bell peppers, diced
- Onion, chopped
- Garlic, minced
- Taco seasoning

Instructions:

1. Brown ground turkey in a skillet.

2. Add diced sweet potatoes, bell peppers, onion,
   and garlic.

3. Season with taco seasoning and cook until sweet
   potatoes are tender.

Prep Time: *25 minutes*

Turkey is a lean protein source, and sweet potatoes offer complex carbohydrates.

Mushroom and Spinach Stuffed Chicken Breast

Ingredients:

- Chicken breast
- Mushrooms, sliced
- Fresh spinach leaves
- Garlic, minced
- Olive oil
- Balsamic glaze

Instructions:

1. Sauté mushrooms, spinach, and minced garlic in olive oil.

2. Cut a pocket in the chicken breast and stuff with the sautéed mixture.

3. Bake until chicken is cooked. Drizzle with balsamic glaze before serving.

Prep Time: *30 minutes*

Chicken provides lean protein, while mushrooms and spinach offer vitamins and minerals.

Lentil and Vegetable Stir-Fry with Tofu

Ingredients:

- Cooked lentils
- Tofu, cubed
- Broccoli florets
- Carrots, sliced
- Soy sauce
- Sesame oil

1. Stir-fry tofu, broccoli, and carrots in sesame oil.

2. Add cooked lentils and soy sauce.

3. Cook until vegetables are tender.

Prep Time: *25 minutes*

Lentils and tofu offer plant-based protein, and vegetables provide essential nutrients.

Egg Fried Cauliflower Rice with Shrimp

Ingredients:

- Cauliflower rice
- Shrimp, peeled and deveined
- Peas and carrots, diced
- Eggs, beaten
- Soy sauce
- Green onions, chopped

Instructions:

1. Sauté shrimp, peas, and carrots in a pan.

2. Push ingredients to one side and scramble eggs on the other side.

3. Add cauliflower rice and soy sauce. Stir to combine.

4. Garnish with chopped green onions.

Prep Time: *20 minutes*

Cauliflower rice is low in carbs, and shrimp provides lean protein.

Chickpea and Vegetable Curry

Ingredients:

- Chickpeas (canned or cooked)
- Mixed vegetables (bell peppers, cauliflower, peas)
- Coconut milk
- Curry powder
- Onion, chopped
- Basmati rice

1. Sauté chopped onion and mixed vegetables in a pot.

2. Add chickpeas, coconut milk, and curry powder.

3. Simmer until vegetables are cooked. Serve over basmati rice.

Prep Time: *30 minutes*

Chickpeas offer plant-based protein, and coconut milk adds healthy fats.

Stuffed Portobello Mushrooms with Quinoa and Feta

Ingredients:

- Portobello mushrooms, cleaned and stems removed
- Cooked quinoa
- Feta cheese
- Cherry tomatoes, diced
- Fresh basil, chopped

- Balsamic glaze

Instructions:

1. Mix cooked quinoa, feta, cherry tomatoes, and fresh basil.
2. Stuff the Portobello mushrooms with the mixture.
3. Bake until mushrooms are tender. Drizzle with balsamic glaze before serving.

Prep Time: *25 minutes*

Quinoa provides complete protein, and Portobello mushrooms offer a hearty base.

Sesame Ginger Tofu Stir-Fry with Brown Rice

Ingredients:

- Tofu, cubed
- Broccoli florets
- Bell peppers, sliced
- Brown rice, cooked

- Soy sauce

- Sesame oil

- Fresh ginger, grated

Instructions:

1. Sauté tofu, broccoli, and bell peppers in sesame oil.

2. Add cooked brown rice, soy sauce, and grated ginger.

3. Stir-fry until heated through.

Prep Time: *25 minutes*

Tofu provides plant-based protein, and brown rice offers complex carbohydrates.

Cauliflower Alfredo with Grilled Chicken

Ingredients:

- Cauliflower, chopped

- Chicken breast, grilled and sliced

- Garlic, minced

- Almond milk
- Nutritional yeast
- Whole-grain fettuccine pasta

Instructions:

1. Boil cauliflower until tender. Blend with almond milk, garlic, and nutritional

2. User

3. Cook whole-grain fettuccine pasta according to package instructions.

4. In a pan, combine the cauliflower Alfredo sauce with the cooked pasta.

5. Top with grilled and sliced chicken breast.

Prep Time: *30 minutes*

Cauliflower provides a low-calorie Alfredo alternative, and grilled chicken offers lean protein.

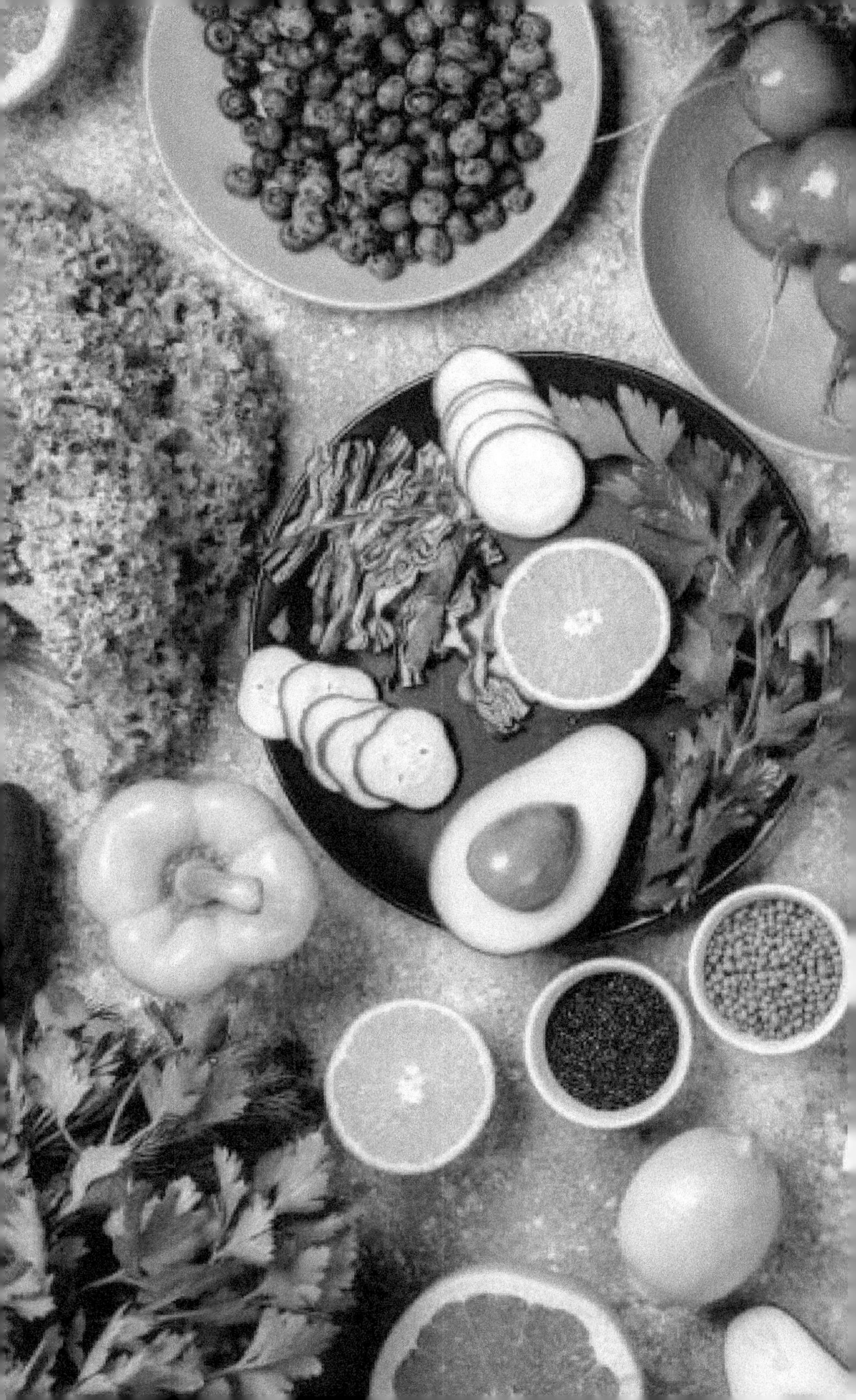

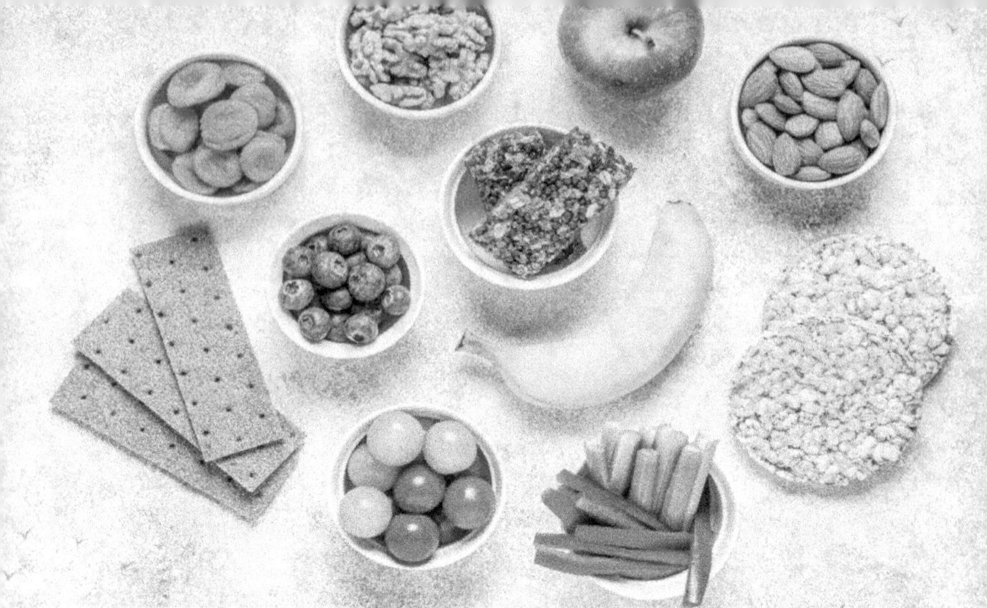

CHAPTER 6: DELICIOUS SNACKS AND TREATS

Greek Yogurt Parfait with Berries and Almonds

Ingredients:

- Greek yogurt
- Mixed berries (blueberries, strawberries)
- Almonds, sliced
- Honey

Instructions:

1. Layer Greek yogurt with mixed berries in a glass.

2. Sprinkle sliced almonds on top.

3. Drizzle with honey before serving.

Prep Time: *5 minutes*

Greek yogurt provides protein and probiotics, while berries and almonds offer antioxidants and healthy fats.

Cucumber and Hummus Bites

Ingredients:

- Cucumber, sliced
- Hummus
- Cherry tomatoes, halved
- Fresh parsley, chopped

Instructions:

1. Top cucumber slices with hummus.

2. Place a halved cherry tomato on each.

3. Garnish with chopped fresh parsley.

Prep Time: 10 minutes

Cucumbers are hydrating, hummus offers plant-based protein, and tomatoes add vitamins.

Energy-Boosting Trail Mix

Ingredients:

- Almonds
- Walnuts
- Dark chocolate chips
- Dried cranberries
- Pumpkin seeds

Instructions:

1. Mix almonds, walnuts, dark chocolate chips, dried cranberries, and pumpkin seeds in a bowl.
2. Portion into snack-sized servings.

Prep Time: *5 minutes*

Nuts provide healthy fats and protein, while dark chocolate and cranberries offer antioxidants.

Apple Slices with Almond Butter

Ingredients:

- Apple, sliced
- Almond butter

Instructions:

1. Spread almond butter on apple slices.
2. Arrange on a plate for a quick and satisfying snack.

Prep Time: *5 minutes*

Apples offer fiber, while almond butter provides healthy fats and protein.

Coconut and Almond Bliss Balls

Ingredients:

- Almond flour

- Shredded coconut
- Dates, pitted
- Almond butter
- Vanilla extract

Instructions:

1. Blend almond flour, shredded coconut, pitted dates, almond butter, and vanilla extract in a food processor.
2. Roll into small balls and refrigerate.

Prep Time: *15 minutes*

Almond flour and almond butter offer healthy fats and protein, while dates provide natural sweetness.

Chia Seed Pudding with Mango

Ingredients:

- Chia seeds
- Almond milk
- Mango, diced

- Coconut flakes

Instructions:

1. Mix chia seeds and almond milk in a jar. Refrigerate overnight.
2. Top with diced mango and coconut flakes before serving.

Prep Time: *5 minutes (plus chilling time)*
Chia seeds offer omega-3 fatty acids and fiber, while mango adds natural sweetness.

Yogurt-Dipped Strawberries

Ingredients:

- Strawberries
- Greek yogurt
- Dark chocolate, melted (optional)

Instructions:

1. Dip strawberries in Greek yogurt.

2. Place on a tray and freeze. Optionally, drizzle with melted dark chocolate.

Prep Time: *10 minutes (plus freezing time) Strawberries provide vitamins, and Greek yogurt offers protein and probiotics.*

Avocado and Tomato Salsa

Ingredients:

- Avocado, diced
- Tomatoes, diced
- Red onion, finely chopped
- Cilantro, chopped
- Lime juice
- Whole-grain tortilla chips

Instructions:

1. Mix diced avocado, tomatoes, red onion, and cilantro.

2. Drizzle with lime juice and serve with whole-grain tortilla chips.

Prep Time: *10 minutes*

Avocado offers healthy fats, and tomatoes add vitamins and antioxidants.

Frozen Banana Bites

Ingredients:

- Bananas, sliced
- Almond butter
- Dark chocolate, melted

Instructions:

1. Spread almond butter between banana slices.
2. Dip in melted dark chocolate and freeze.

Prep Time: *15 minutes (plus freezing time)*

Bananas provide potassium, and almond butter offers healthy fats and protein.

Pumpkin Spice Smoothie Bowl

Ingredients:

- Frozen banana
- Pumpkin puree
- Greek yogurt
- Almond milk
- Pumpkin spice
- Granola and sliced almonds for topping

Instructions:

1. Blend frozen banana, pumpkin puree, Greek yogurt, almond milk, and pumpkin spice until smooth.
2. Pour into a bowl and top with granola and sliced almonds.

Prep Time: *10 minutes*

Pumpkin provides vitamins, and Greek yogurt offers protein and probiotics.

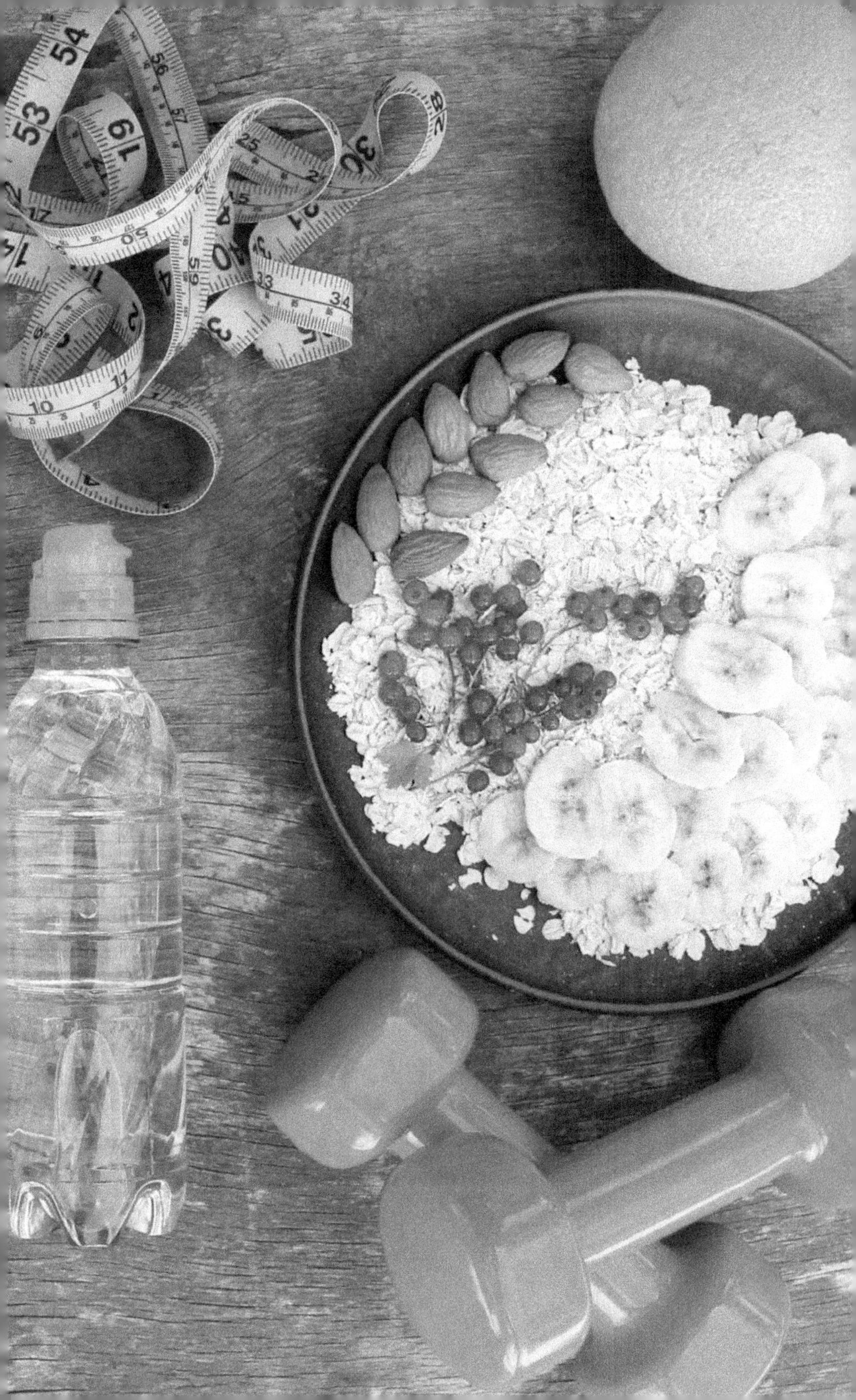

30-Day Meal Planning Challenge

Month

Meal Plan Schedule

DAY 1	DAY 2	DAY 3	DAY 4	DAY 5
DAY	DAY 7	DAY 8	DAY 9	DAY 10
DAY 11	DAY 12	DAY 13	DAY 14	DAY 15
DAY 16	DAY 17	DAY 18	DAY 19	DAY 20
DAY 21	DAY 22	DAY 23	DAY 24	DAY 25
DAY 26	DAY 27	DAY 28	DAY 29	DAY 30

WEEK:

GROCERIES LIST

BREAKFAST	LUNCH	DINNER	
			MONDAY
			TUESDAY
			WEDNESDAY
			THURSDAY
			FRIDAY
			SATURDAY
			SUNDAY

WEEK:

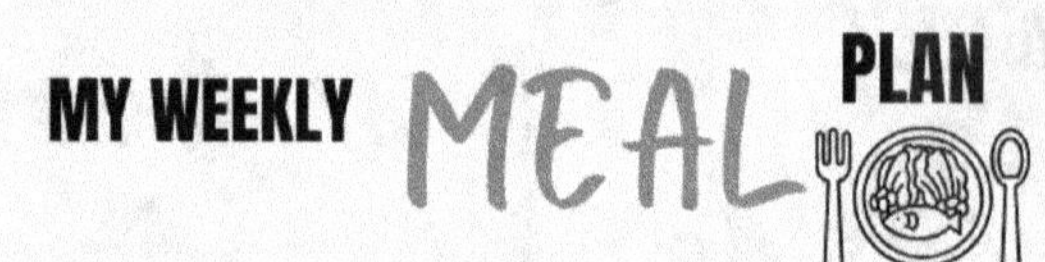

MEAL PLAN SCHEDULE

SNACKS

DRINKS

FRUITS

VEGETABLES

RECIPES

DATE: ______________

Recipe Name

- [ ] Lean proteins
- [ ] Whole grains
- [ ] Healthy fats
- [ ] Vegetables
- [ ] Fruits

Prep Time

Cooking Time

Serve

Notes

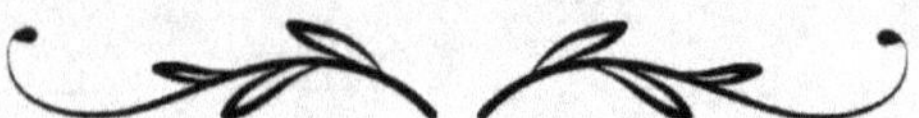

Personal *Journal*

Date:...........................

1	2	3	4	5	6
				MEETING	
7	8	9	10	11	12
13	14	15	16	17	18
19	20	21	22	23	24
25	26	27	28	29	30
		DON'T 4GET			

Note

Habit Tracker

Workout

Yoga

Eat Clean

Describe your initial thoughts and feelings about incorporating fasting into your lifestyle. How has your perception changed over time?

____

____

____

Record your energy levels throughout the day during fasting periods. What patterns do you notice, and how do they correlate with your fasting routine?

____

____

____

____

Share and reflect on your go-to recipes that align with the principles of fasting. How do these meals contribute to your overall well-being?

____

____

____

____

WEEK:

GROCERIES LIST

MY WEEKLY MEAL PLAN

BREAKFAST	LUNCH	DINNER

MONDAY

TUESDAY

WEDNESDAY

THURSDAY

FRIDAY

SATURDAY

SUNDAY

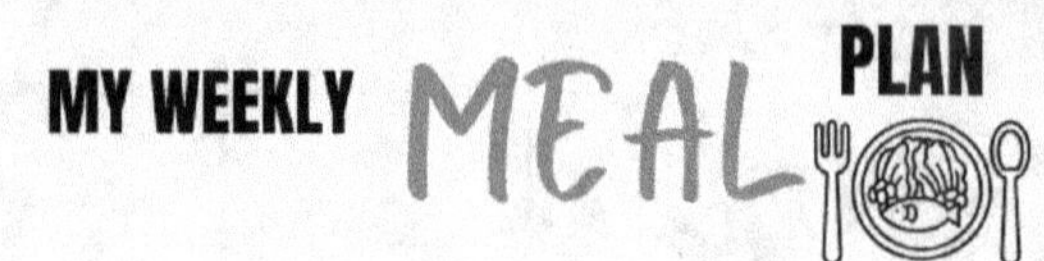

MEAL PLAN SCHEDULE

SNACKS

DRINKS

FRUITS

VEGETABLES

RECIPES

DATE: ______

Recipe Name

- Lean proteins
- Whole grains
- Healthy fats
- Vegetables
- Fruits

Prep Time

Cooking Time

Serve

Notes

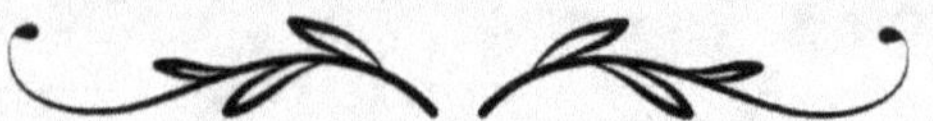

Personal *Journal*

Date:........................

1	2	3	4	5 MEETING	6
7	8	9	10	11	12
13	14	15	16	17	18
19	20	21	22	23	24
25	26	27 DON'T 4GET	28	29	30

Note

....
....
....
....
....
....
....
....
....
....

Habit Tracker

Workout

Yoga

Eat Clean

Monitor and journal any changes in your hormonal balance since starting the fasting journey. How have these changes positively impacted your life?

____

____

____

____

Explore moments of mindful eating during and after fasting periods. How has incorporating mindfulness into your meals enhanced your overall experience?

____

____

____

____

Document your exercise routine alongside your fasting schedule. What physical activities complement your fasting journey, and how do they contribute to your well-being?

____

____

____

WEEK:

GROCERIES LIST

MY WEEKLY MEAL PLAN

	BREAKFAST	LUNCH	DINNER
MONDAY			
TUESDAY			
WEDNESDAY			
THURSDAY			
FRIDAY			
SATURDAY			
SUNDAY			

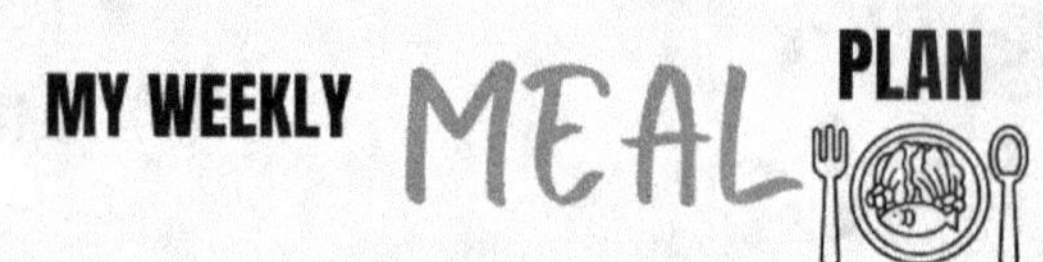

MEAL PLAN SCHEDULE

SNACKS

DRINKS

FRUITS

VEGETABLES

RECIPES

DATE: ________________

Recipe Name

- [ ] **Lean proteins**
- [ ] **Whole grains**
- [ ] **Healthy fats**
- [ ] **Vegetables**
- [ ] **Fruits**

Prep Time

Cooking Time

Serve

Notes

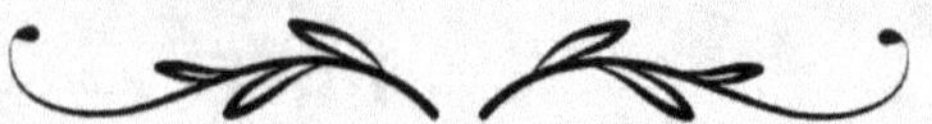

Personal *Journal*

Date:...................

1	2	3	4	5	6
				MEETiNG	
7	8	9	10	11	12
13	14	15	16	17	18
19	20	21	22	23	24
25	26	27	28	29	30
		DON'T 4GET			

Note

Habit Tracker

Workout

Yoga

Eat Clean

Describe the self-care practices you engage in during fasting periods. How do these rituals support your mental and emotional well-being?

____

____

____

____

Experiment with different fasting schedules (e.g., intermittent fasting, extended fasting). What variations work best for you, and how do they impact your health goals?

____

____

____

____

Reflect on the challenges you've faced during your fasting journey and celebrate the triumphs. How have these experiences shaped your relationship with fasting?

____

____

____

____

GROCERIES
LIST

MY WEEKLY MEAL PLAN

	BREAKFAST	LUNCH	DINNER
MONDAY			
TUESDAY			
WEDNESDAY			
THURSDAY			
FRIDAY			
SATURDAY			
SUNDAY			

MY WEEKLY 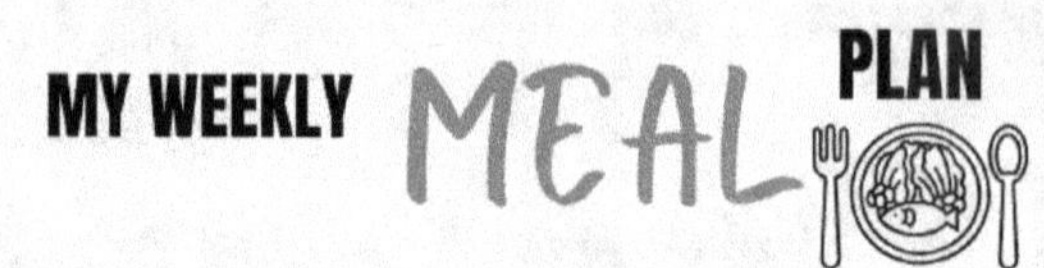

MEAL PLAN SCHEDULE

SNACKS

DRINKS

FRUITS

VEGETABLES

RECIPES

DATE: ______________

Recipe Name

- [ ] Lean proteins
- [ ] Whole grains
- [ ] Healthy fats
- [ ] Vegetables
- [ ] Fruits

Prep Time

Cooking Time

Serve

Notes

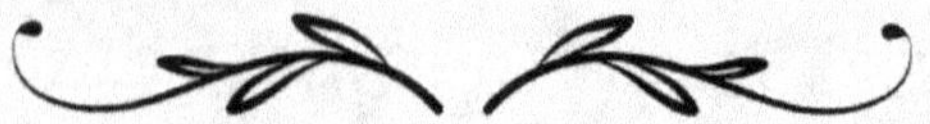

Personal *Journal*

Date:..........................

1	2	3	4	5	6
				MEETING	
7	8	9	10	11	12
13	14	15	16	17	18
19	20	21	22	23	24
25	26	27	28	29	30
		DON'T 4GET			

Note

....
....
....
....
....
....
....
....
....
....
....
....

Habit Tracker

Workout

Yoga

Eat Clean

Experiment with different fasting schedules (e.g., intermittent fasting, extended fasting). What variations work best for you, and how do they impact your health goals?

____

____

____

____

Consider the influence of social and cultural factors on your fasting journey. How do you navigate social events and cultural practices while fasting?

____

____

____

____

Reflect on your perception of body image throughout the fasting process. How has fasting influenced your relationship with your body, and what positive changes have you noticed?

____

____

____

____

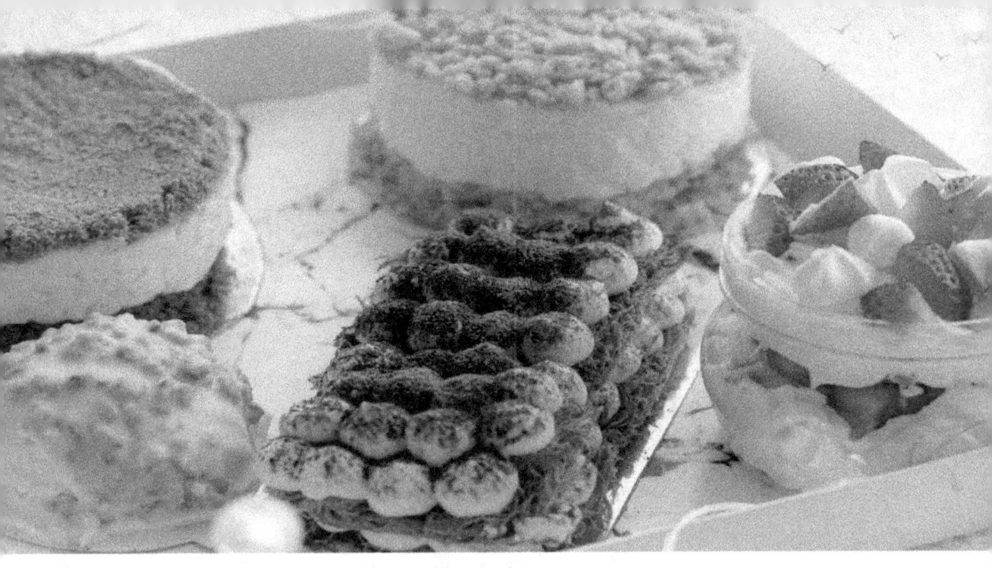

CHAPTER 8: DELICIOUS DESSERT

Chocolate Avocado Mousse

Ingredients:

- Ripe avocados
- Cocoa powder
- Maple syrup or honey
- Vanilla extract

Instructions:

1. Blend avocados, cocoa powder, maple syrup (or honey), and vanilla extract until smooth.

2. Chill in the refrigerator before serving.

Prep Time: *10 minutes*

Avocados provide healthy fats, and cocoa is rich in antioxidants.

Berry and Yogurt Parfait

Ingredients:

- Mixed berries (strawberries, blueberries, raspberries)
- Greek yogurt
- Granola
- Honey

Instructions:

1. Layer Greek yogurt, mixed berries, and granola in a glass.
2. Drizzle with honey before serving.

Prep Time: *5 minutes*

Greek yogurt offers protein and probiotics, and berries provide vitamins and antioxidants.

Pumpkin Chia Seed Pudding

Ingredients:

- Chia seeds
- Almond milk
- Pumpkin puree
- Maple syrup
- Pumpkin spice

Instructions:

1. Mix chia seeds, almond milk, pumpkin puree, maple syrup, and pumpkin spice.
2. Refrigerate overnight or until set.

Prep Time: *5 minutes (plus chilling time)*
Chia seeds offer omega-3 fatty acids, and pumpkin provides vitamins and fiber.

Coconut and Almond Flour Brownies

Ingredients:

- Almond flour
- Cocoa powder
- Coconut oil
- Maple syrup
- Eggs
- Dark chocolate chips

Instructions:

1. Mix almond flour, cocoa powder, melted coconut oil, maple syrup, and eggs.
2. Fold in dark chocolate chips and bake until set.

Prep Time: *20 minutes*

Almond flour and coconut oil provide healthy fats, and dark chocolate offers antioxidants.

Mango Sorbet

Ingredients:

- Frozen mango chunks
- Coconut water
- Lime juice
- Mint leaves for garnish

Instructions:

1. Blend frozen mango chunks, coconut water, and lime juice until smooth.
2. Freeze until firm. Garnish with mint leaves before serving.

Prep Time: *10 minutes (plus freezing time)*
Mango provides vitamins, and coconut water offers hydration.

Baked Apples with Cinnamon and Walnuts

Ingredients:

- Apples, cored and sliced
- Cinnamon
- Walnuts, chopped
- Maple syrup

Instructions:

1. Arrange apple slices in a baking dish.
2. Sprinkle with cinnamon, chopped walnuts, and drizzle with maple syrup.
3. Bake until apples are tender.

Prep Time: *15 minutes*

Apples provide fiber, and walnuts offer healthy fats.

Cherry Almond Dark Chocolate Bark

Ingredients:

- Dark chocolate, melted
- Dried cherries
- Almonds, sliced
- Sea salt

1. Spread melted dark chocolate on a parchment-lined tray.

2. Sprinkle with dried cherries, sliced almonds, and sea salt.

3. Refrigerate until set, then break into pieces.

Prep Time: *15 minutes (plus chilling time)*
Dark chocolate provides antioxidants, and almonds offer healthy fats.

Blueberry Lemon Cheesecake Bites

Ingredients:

- Cream cheese
- Blueberries
- Lemon zest
- Vanilla extract
- Graham cracker crumbs for coating

1. Mix cream cheese, blueberries, lemon zest, and vanilla extract.
2. Form into small bites and roll in graham cracker crumbs.

Prep Time: *20 minutes*

Blueberries offer antioxidants, and cream cheese provides a creamy texture.

Banana and Peanut Butter Ice Cream

Ingredients:

- Frozen bananas
- Peanut butter
- Almond milk

Instructions:

1. Blend frozen bananas, peanut butter, and almond milk until smooth.
2. Freeze until scoopable.

Prep Time: *10 minutes (plus freezing time)*

Bananas offer natural sweetness, and peanut butter provides protein and healthy fats.

Lemon Poppy Seed Yogurt Cake

Ingredients:

- Greek yogurt
- Almond flour
- Lemon juice and zest
- Poppy seeds
- Maple syrup
- Eggs

Instructions:

1. Mix Greek yogurt, almond flour, lemon juice, zest, poppy seeds, maple syrup, and eggs.
2. Bake until set.

Prep Time: *30 minutes*

Greek yogurt provides protein and probiotics, and almonds offer healthy fats.

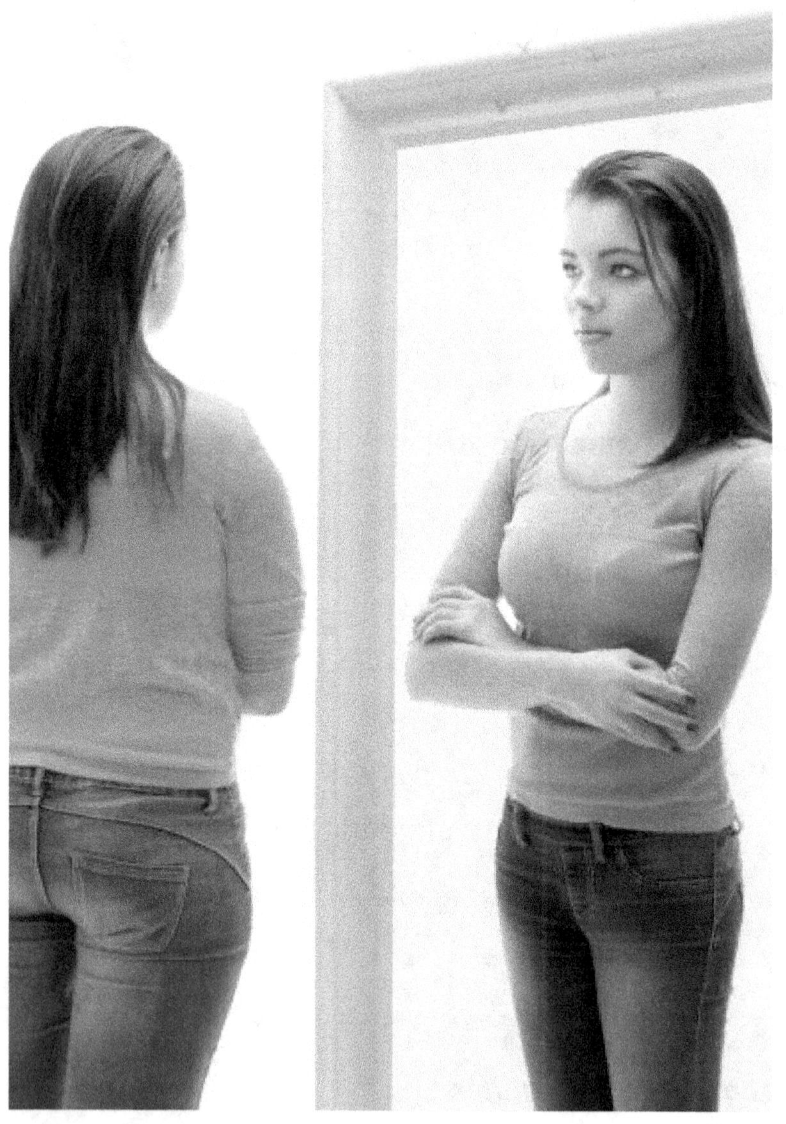

9 7 9 8 8 8 7 5 6 6 3 8 4 0